CW00903712

Other titles in the series:
The Victim's Guide to the Doctor
The Victim's Guide to Middle Age

Published in the USA in 1993 by Exley Giftbooks.
Published in Great Britain in 1993 by Exley Publications Ltd
Reprinted 1993

Cartoons copyright © Roland Fiddy, 1993
Copyright © Exley Publications, 1993

ISBN 1-85015-404-X

A copy of the CIP data is available from the
British Library on request.

Printed in Spain by Grafo, S.A. – Bilbao.

Exley Publications Ltd, 16 Chalk Hill, Watford, Herts WD1 4BN,
United Kingdom.
Exley Giftbooks, 359 East Main Street, Suite 3D, Mount Kisco,
NY 10549, USA.

THE VICTIM'S GUIDE TO ...

The Dentist

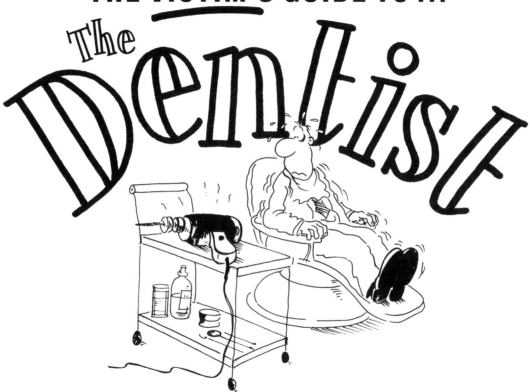

EXLEY

MT. KISCO, NEW YORK • WATFORD, UK

Many people suffer from DENTISTPHOBIA*

* A reluctance to sit in a chair while a person in a white coat sticks needles in your gums, makes holes in your teeth with an electric drill, pulls your teeth out with a pair of pliers, and keeps asking questions which you cannot answer because your mouth is wide open.

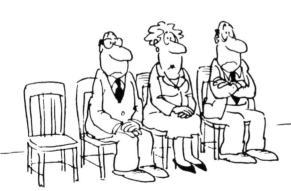
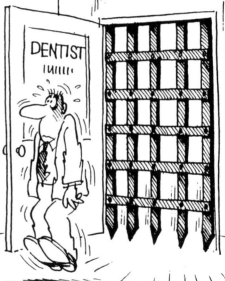

WAITING ROOM

DENTIST

CLANG!!

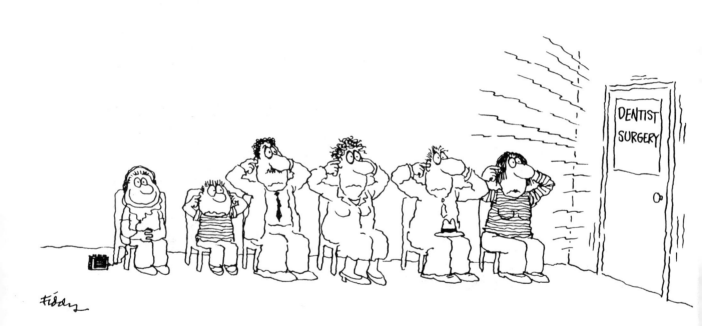

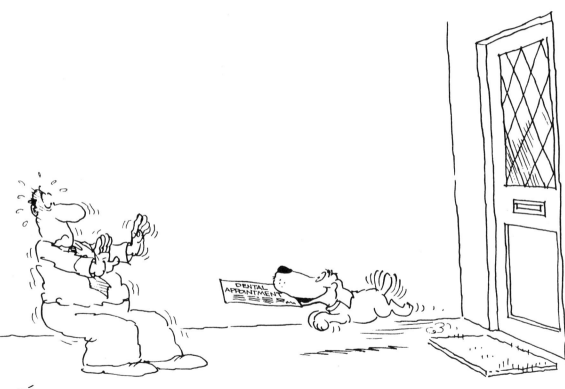

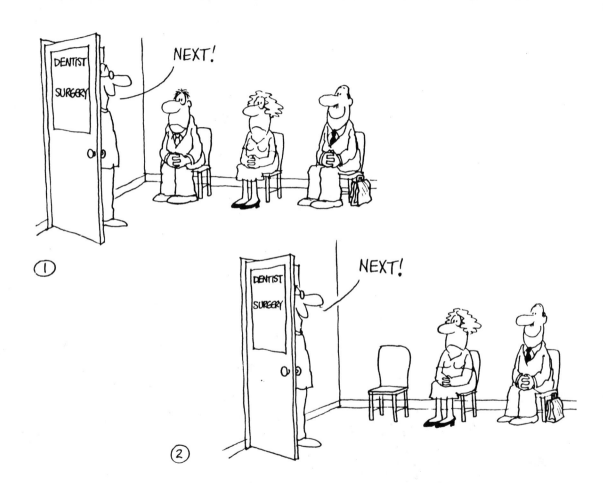

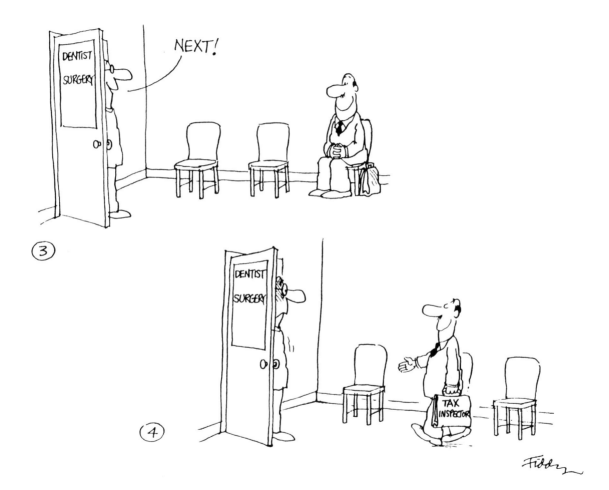

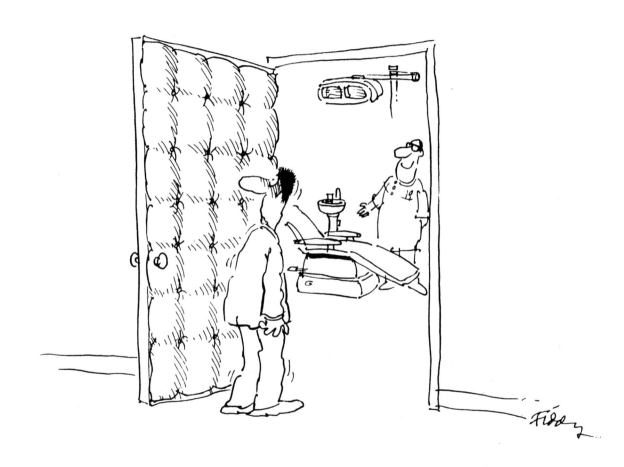

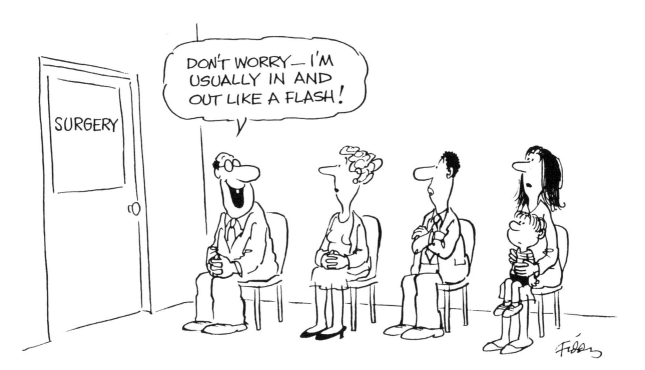

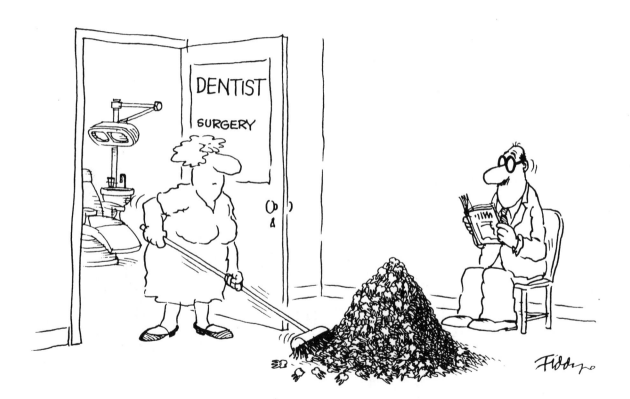

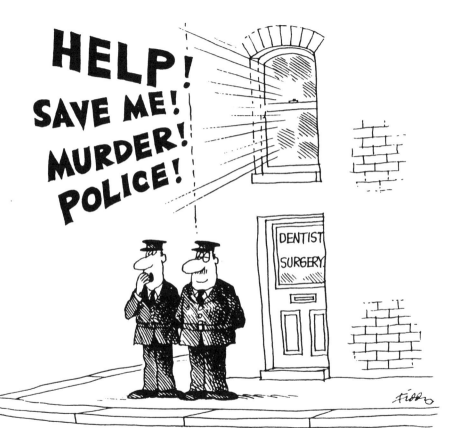

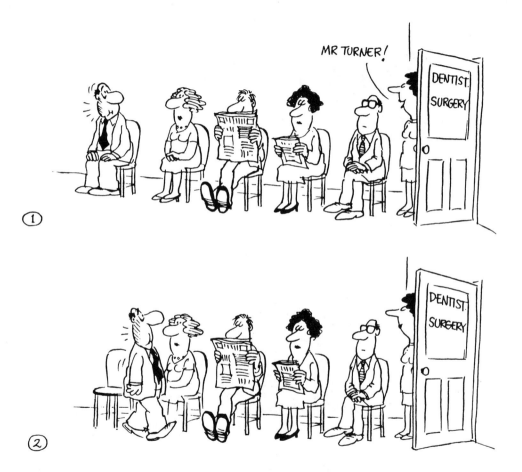

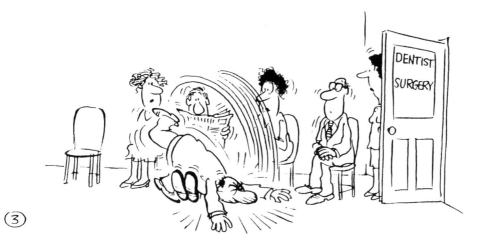

③

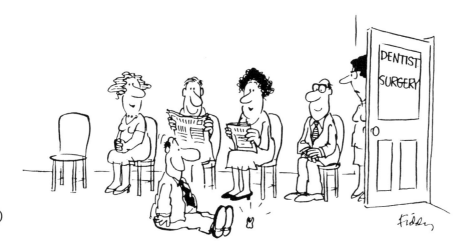

④

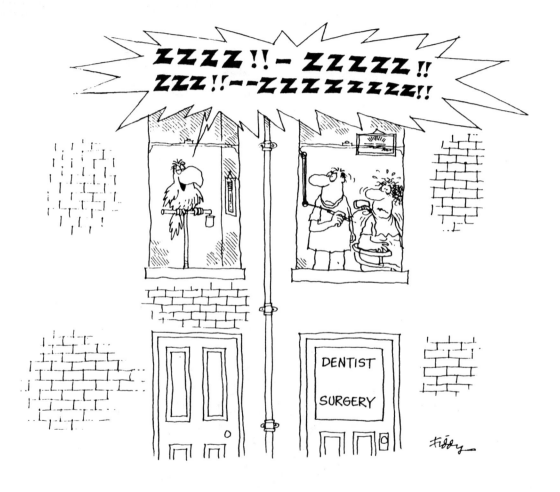

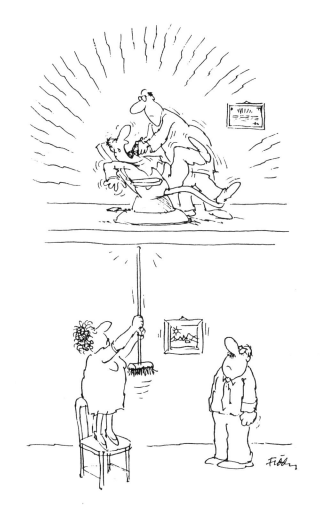

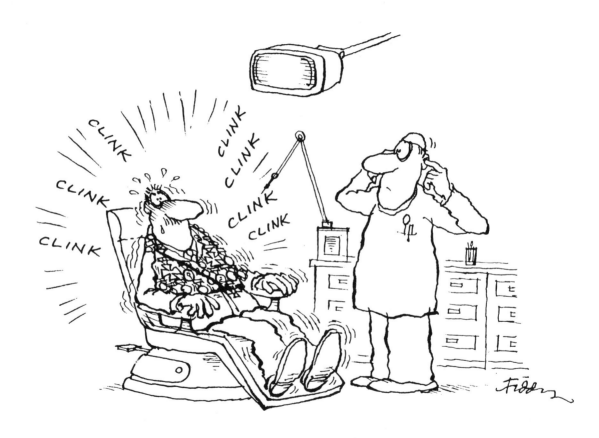

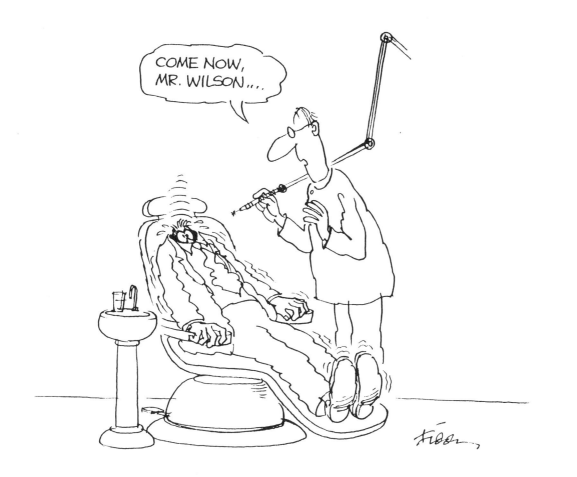

SILENCE PLEASE

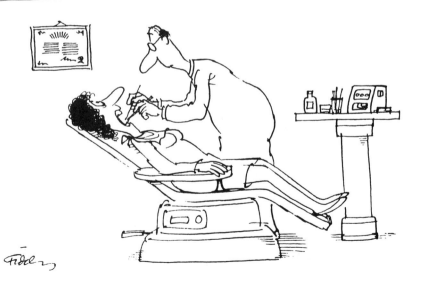

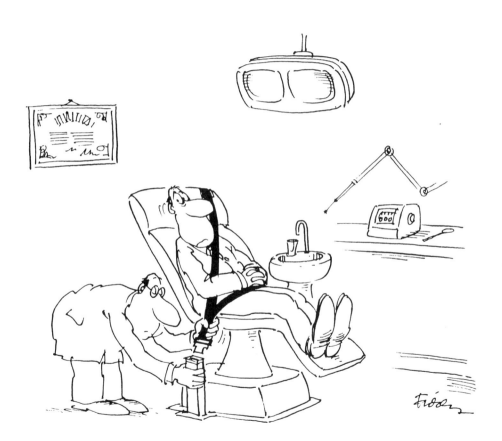

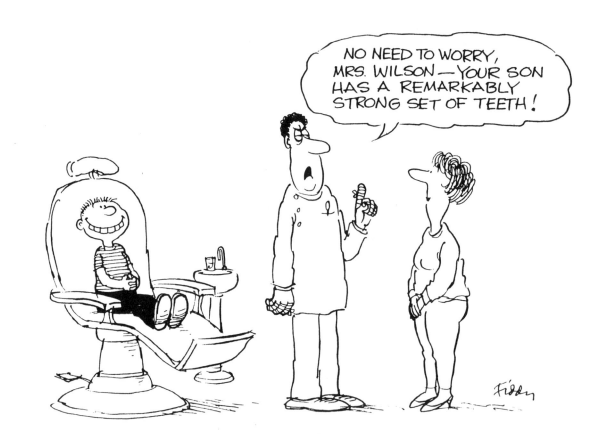

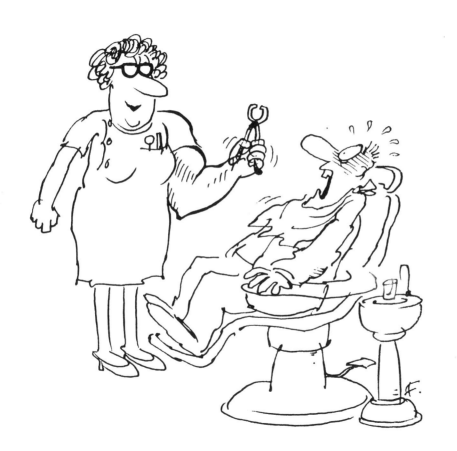

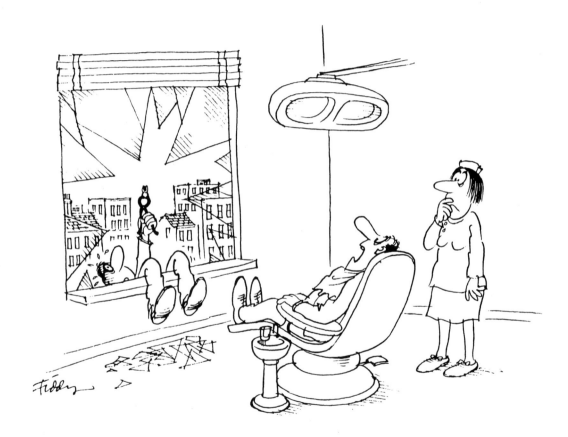

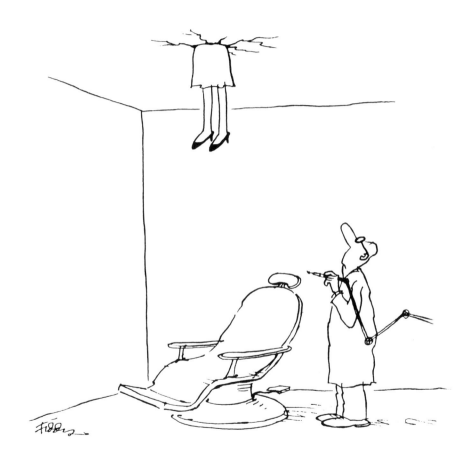

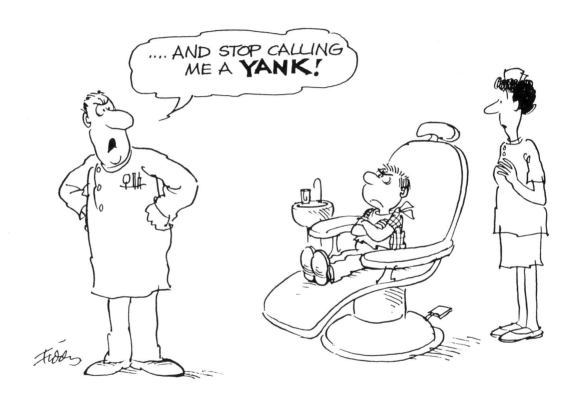

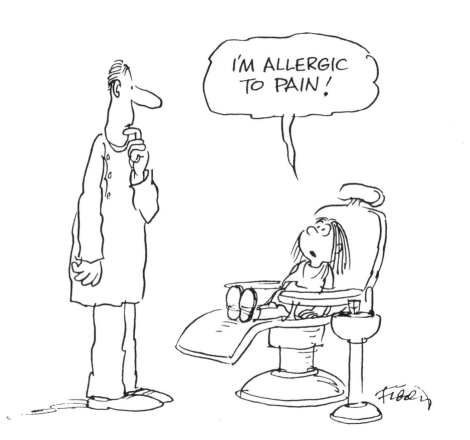

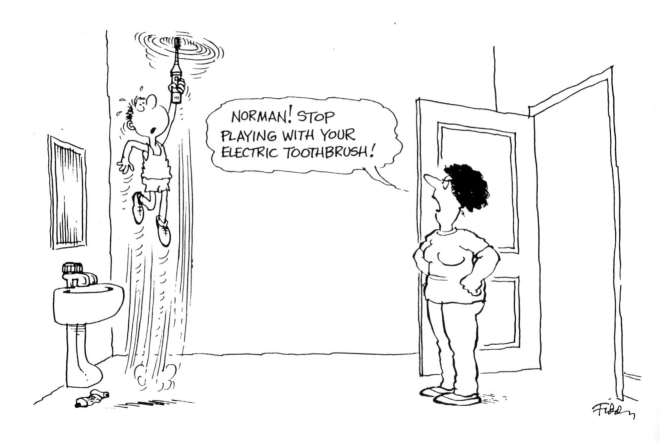

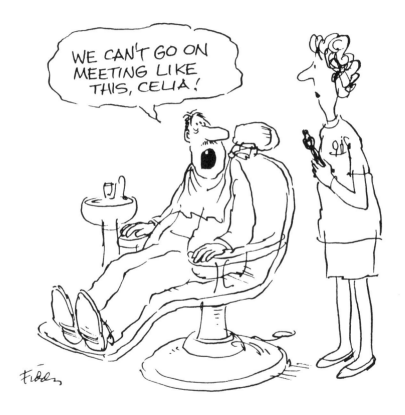

Teeth Encounter.

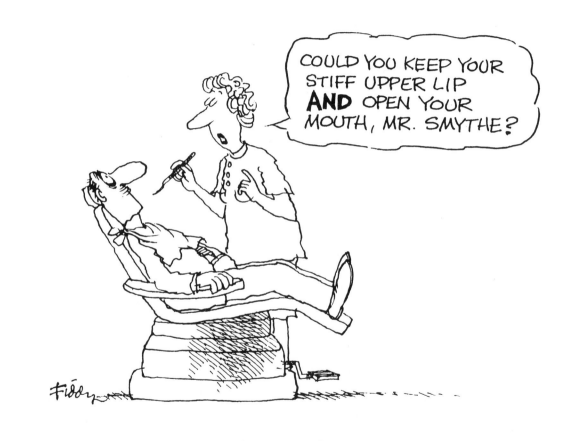

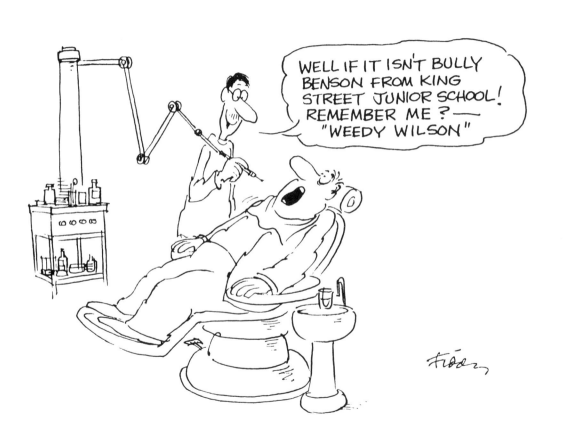

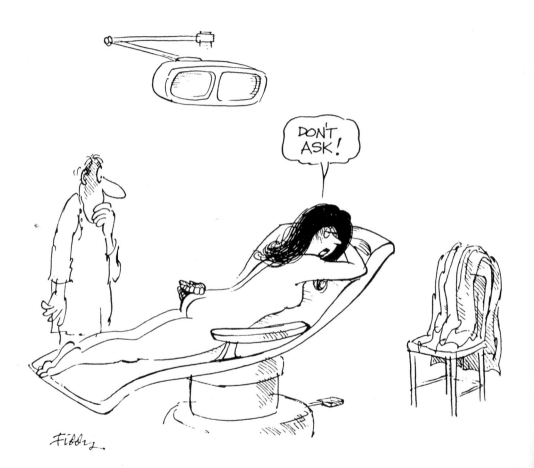

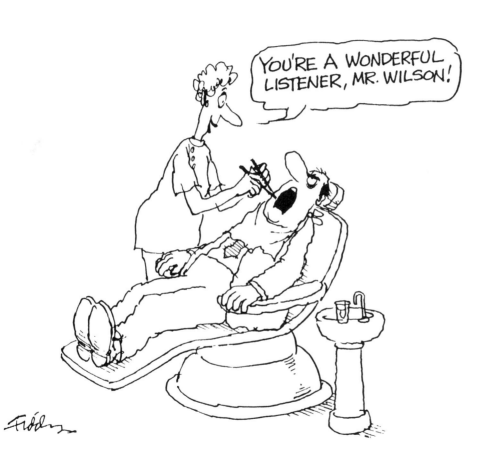

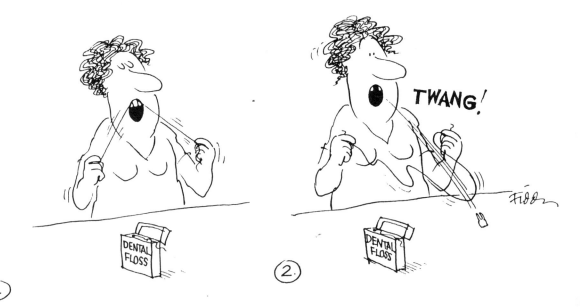

Sometimes, in spite of Preventive Dentistry, people lose their teeth.

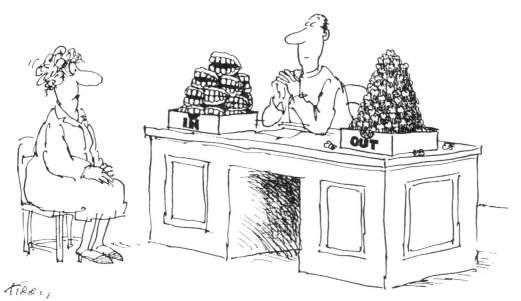

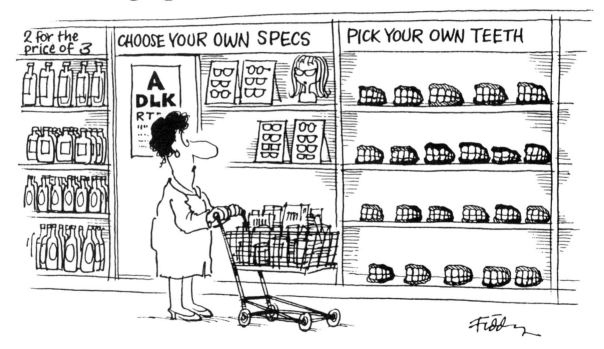

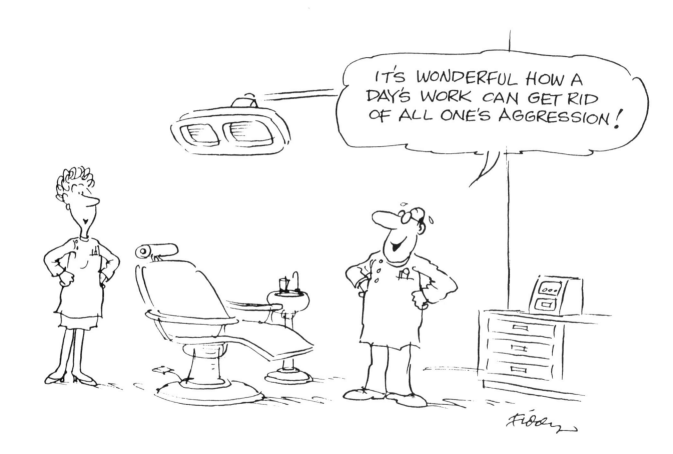

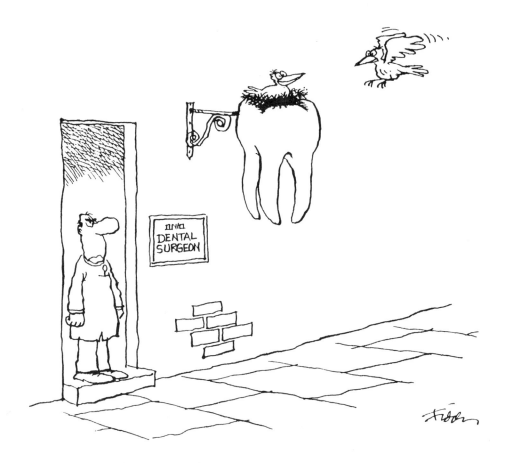

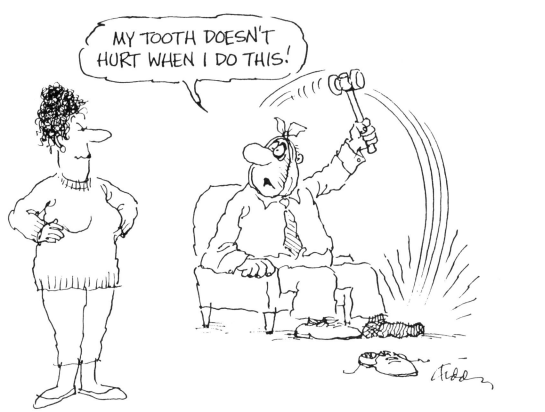

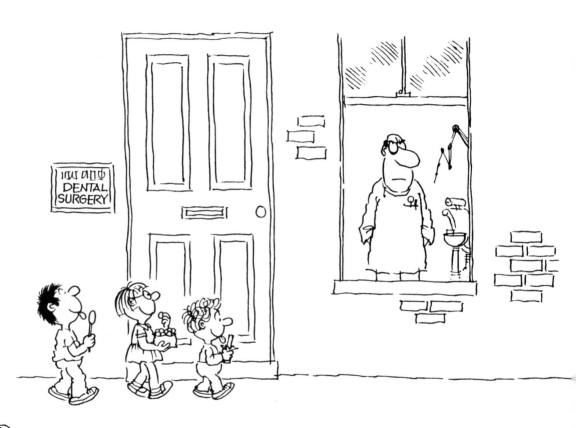

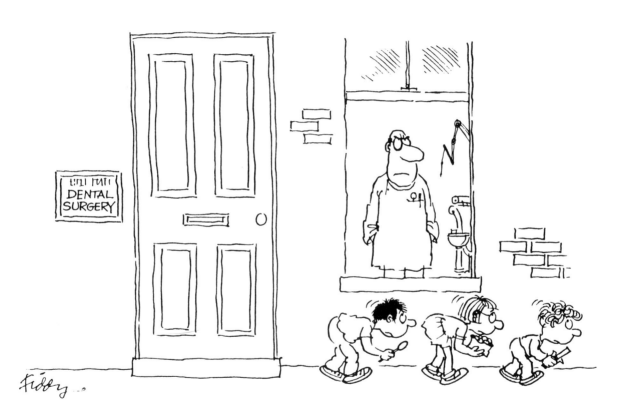

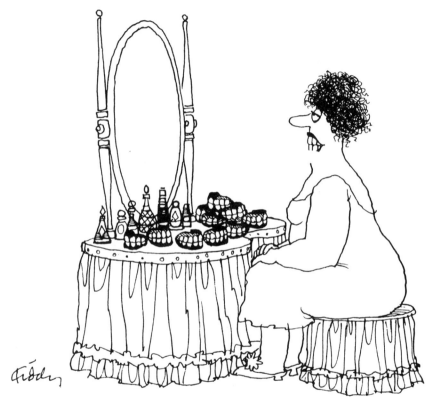

Patients with new dentures often need to return to the dentist for adjustments . . . .

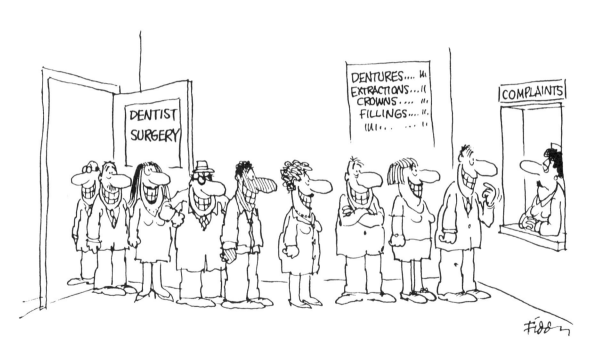

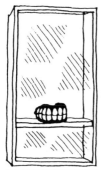

IN CASE OF
EMERGENCY
BREAK GLASS

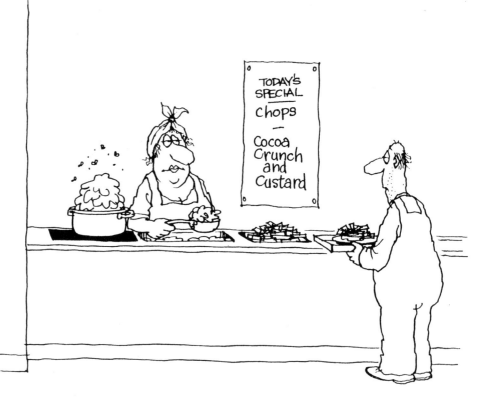

TODAY'S
SPECIAL

Chops
—
Cocoa
Crunch
and
Custard

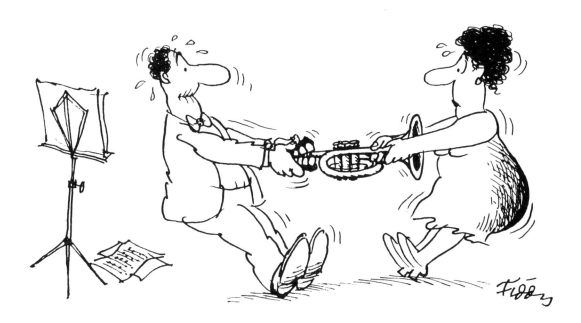

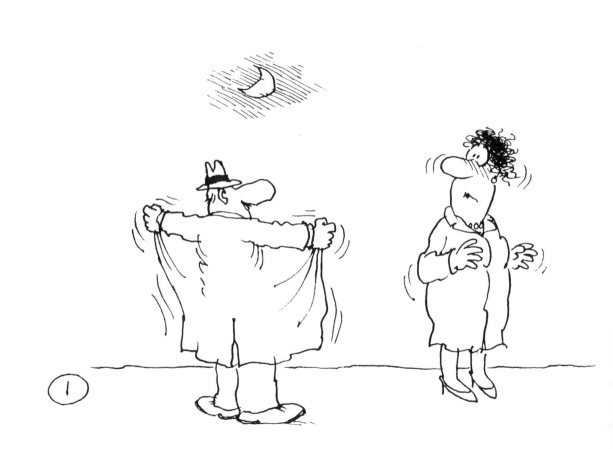

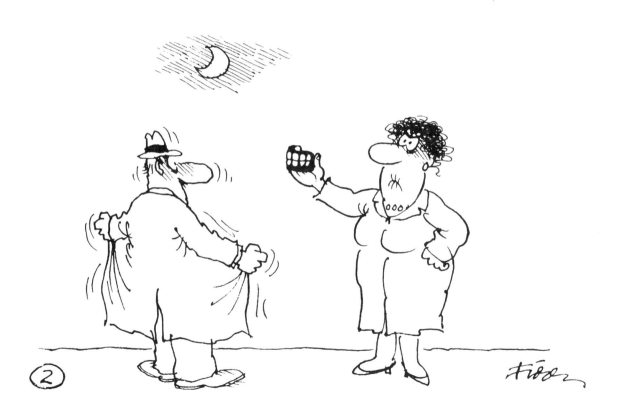

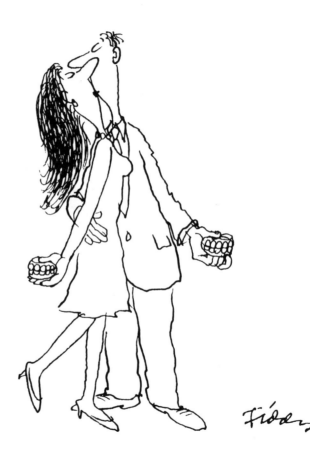

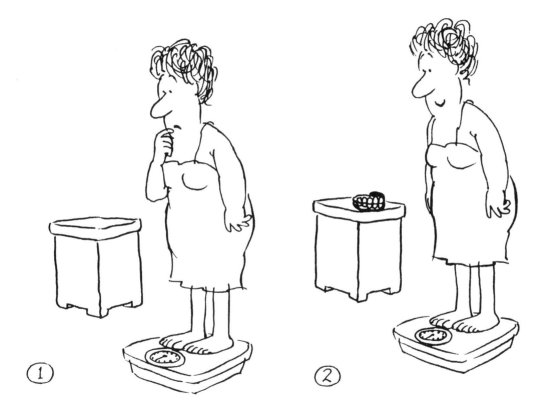

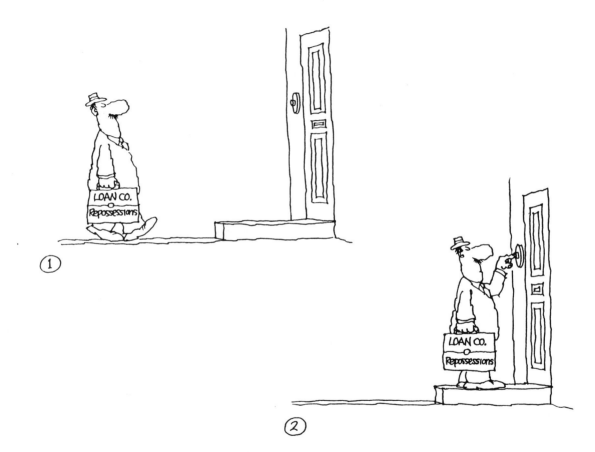

① ②

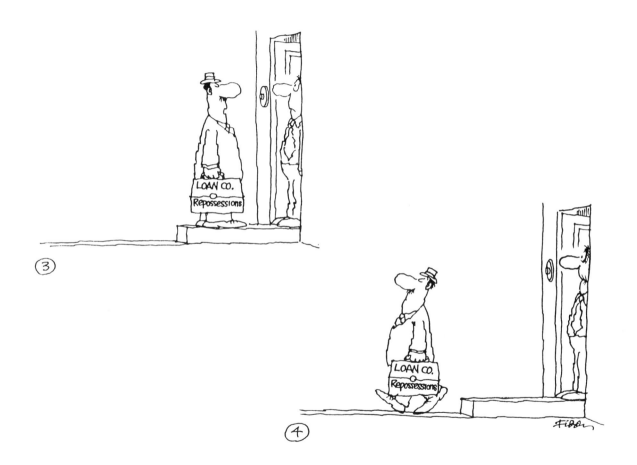

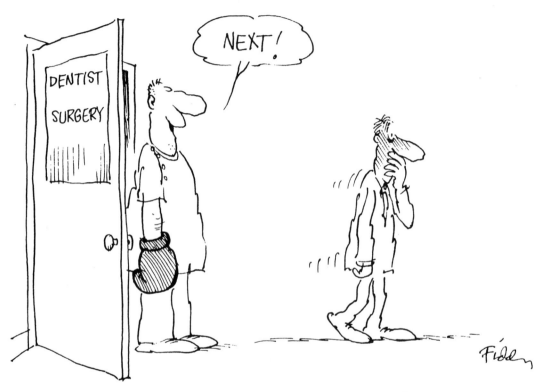

There are good dentists and bad dentists....

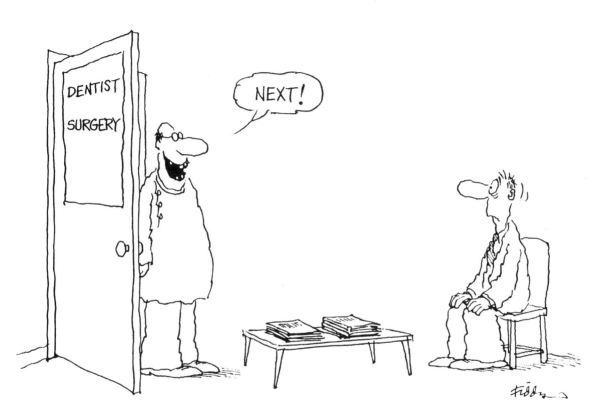

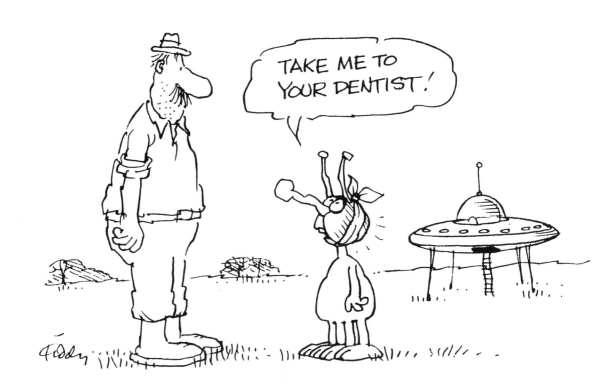

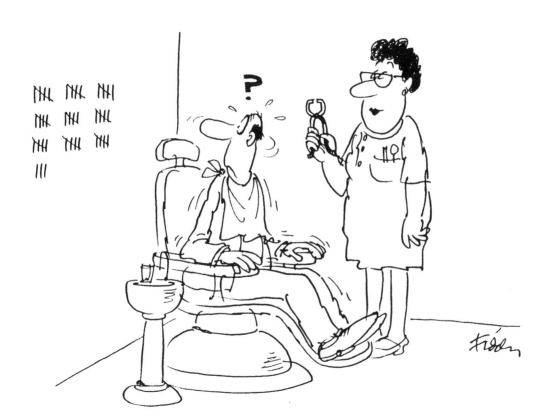

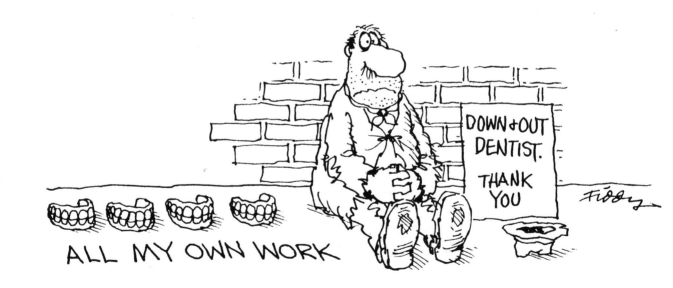

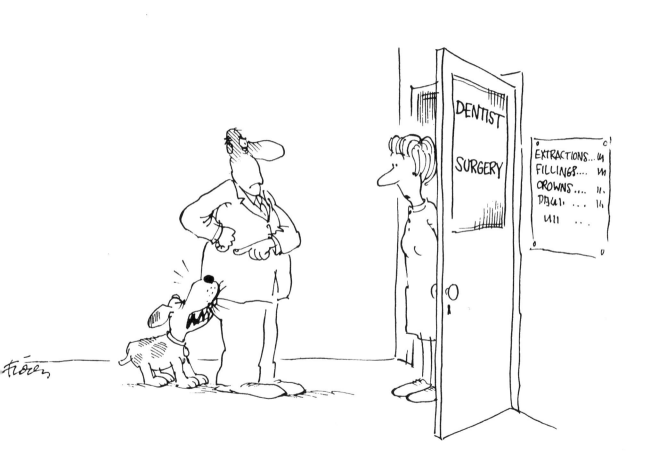

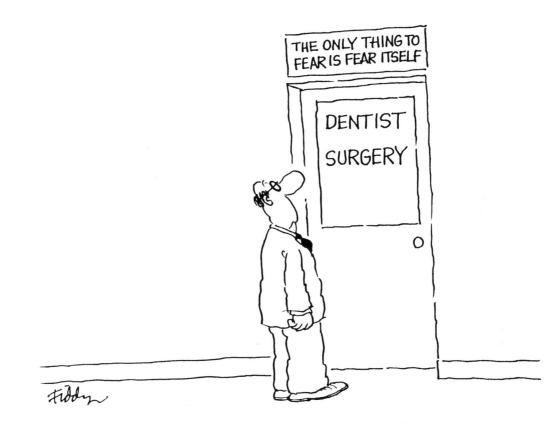

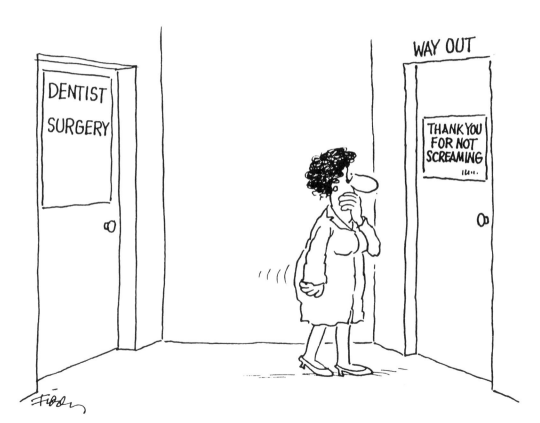

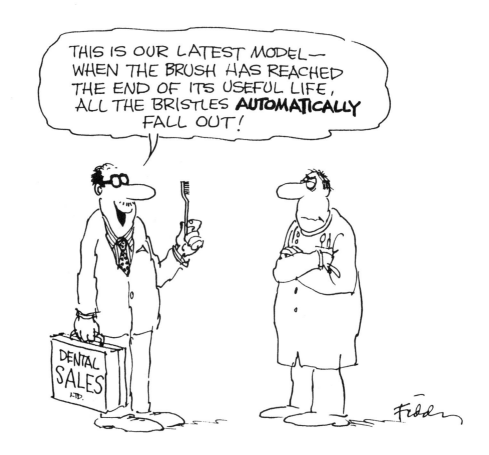

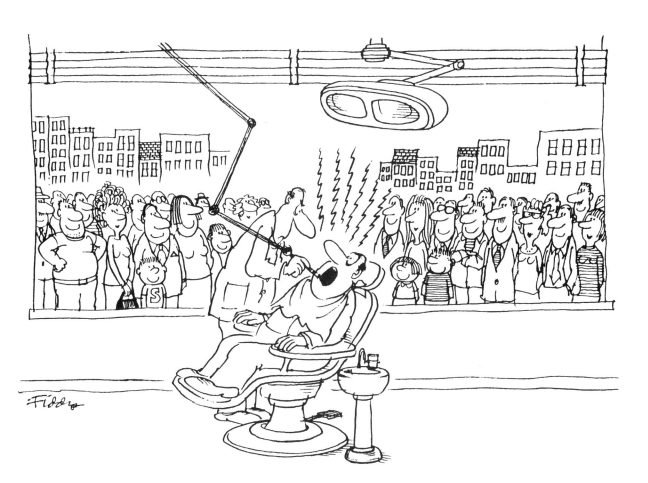

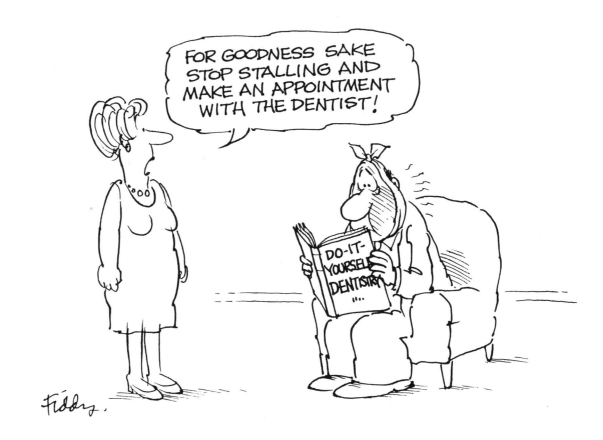

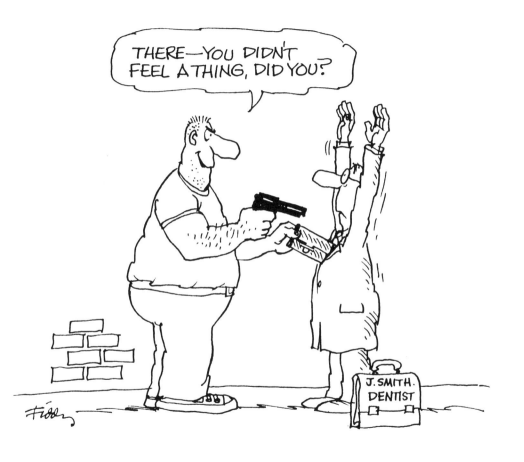

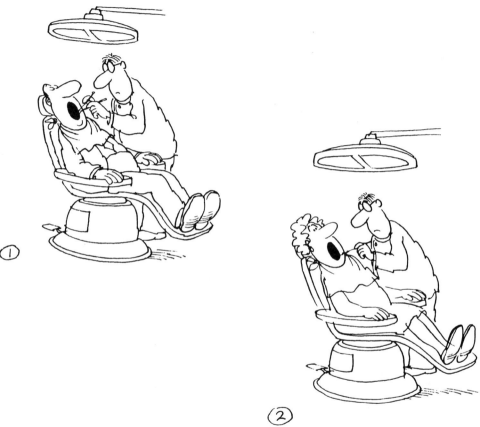

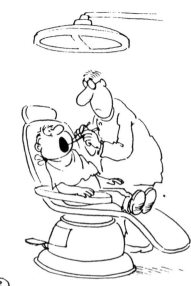

③

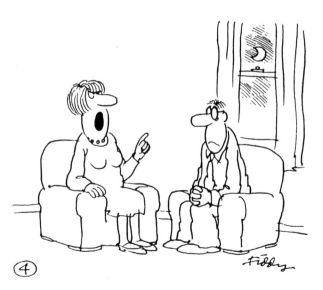

④

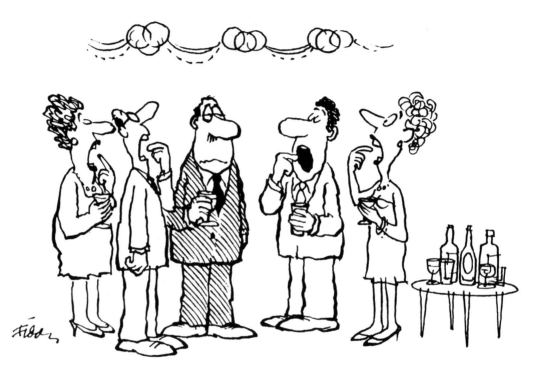

Never forget that when dentists go home they are
human, just like everybody else .....

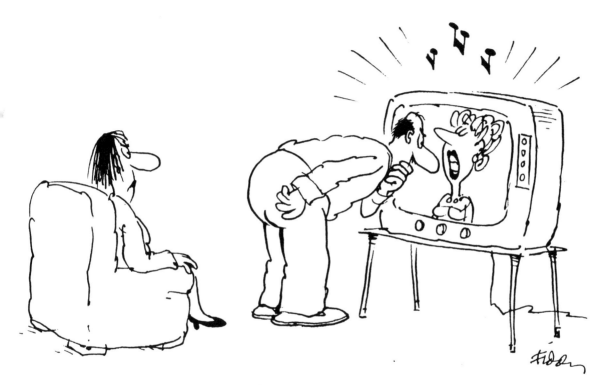

.... well, nearly like everybody else.

The Dentist at Home.

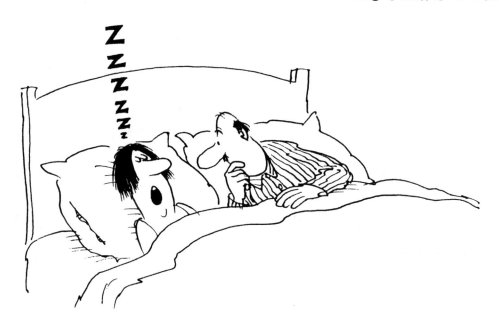

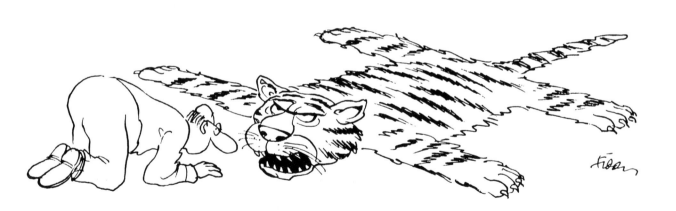

The Dentist at Home.

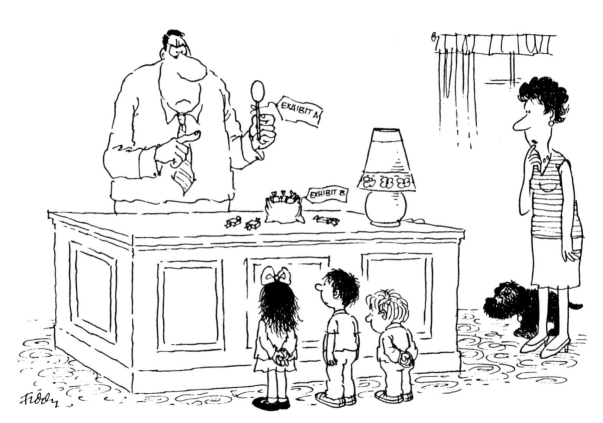

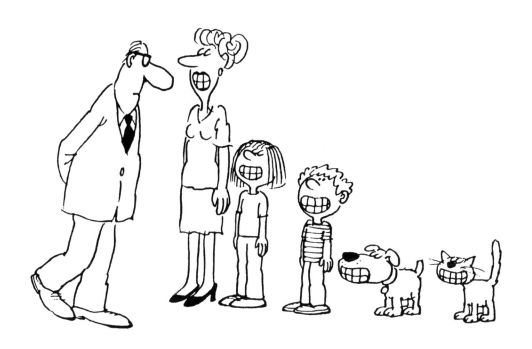

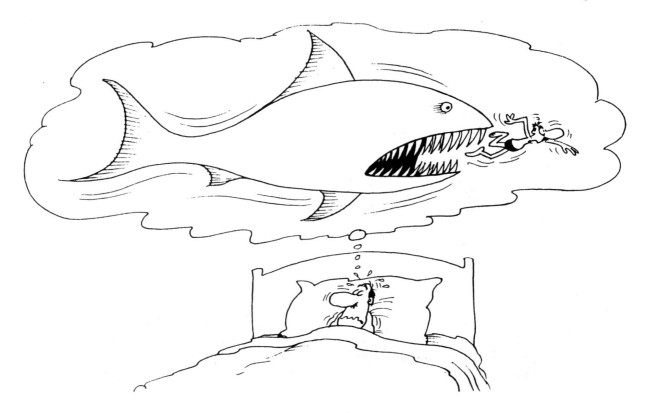

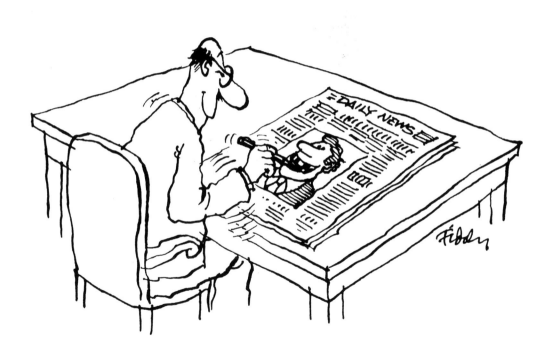

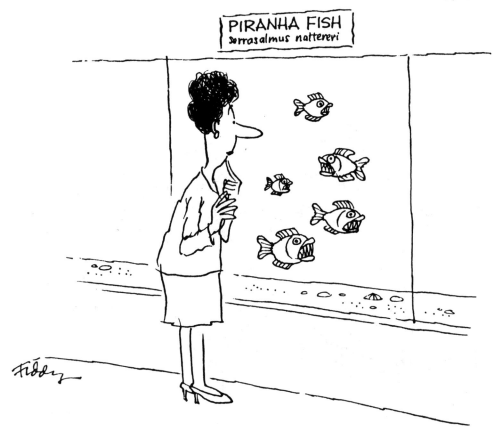

The Dentist at Leisure

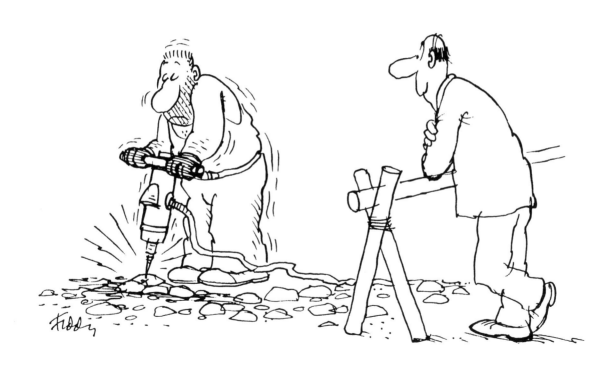

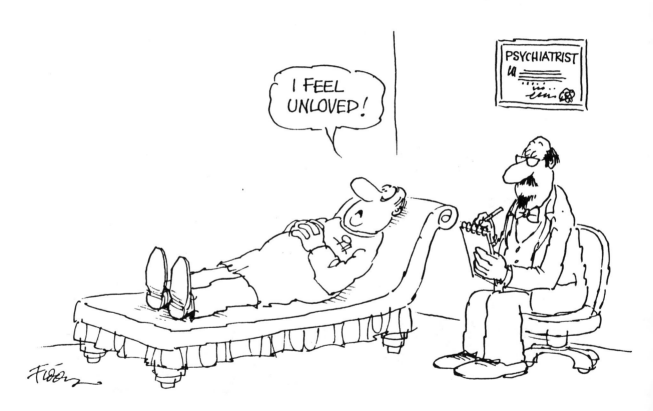

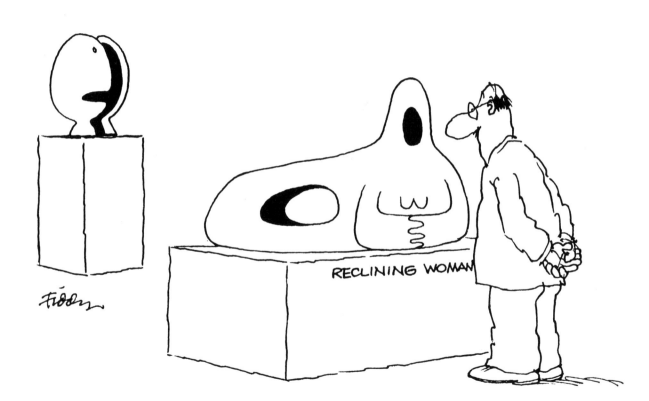

RECLINING WOMAN

Books in the "Crazy World" series
($4.99 £2.99 paperback)

The Crazy World of Aerobics (Bill Stott)
The Crazy World of Cats (Bill Stott)
The Crazy World of Cricket (Bill Stott)
The Crazy World of Gardening (Bill Stott)
The Crazy World of Golf (Mike Scott)
The Crazy World of the Greens (Barry Knowles)
The Crazy World of The Handyman (Roland Fiddy)
The Crazy World of Hospitals (Bill Stott)
The Crazy World of Housework (Bill Stott)
The Crazy World of Learning (Bill Stott)
The Crazy World of Love (Roland Fiddy)
The Crazy World of Marriage (Bill Stott)
The Crazy World of The Office (Bill Stott)
The Crazy World of Photography (Bill Stott)
The Crazy World of Rugby (Bill Stott)
The Crazy World of Sailing (Peter Rigby)
The Crazy World of Sex (David Pye)

Books in the "Mini Joke Book" series
($6.99 £3.99 hardback)

These attractive 64 page mini joke books are illustrated throughout by Bill Stott.

A Binge of Diet Jokes
A Bouquet of Wedding Jokes
A Feast of After Dinner Jokes
A Knockout of Sports Jokes
A Portfolio of Business Jokes
A Round of Golf Jokes
A Romp of Naughty Jokes
A Spread of Over-40s Jokes
A Tankful of Motoring Jokes

Books in the "Fanatics" series
($4.99 £2.99 paperback)

The **Fanatic's Guides** are perfect presents for everyone with a hobby that has got out of hand. Eighty pages of hilarious black and white cartoons by Roland Fiddy.

The Fanatic's Guide to the Bed
The Fanatic's Guide to Cats
The Fanatic's Guide to Computers
The Fanatic's Guide to Dads
The Fanatic's Guide to Diets
The Fanatic's Guide to Dogs
The Fanatic's Guide to Husbands
The Fanatic's Guide to Money
The Fanatic's Guide to Sex
The Fanatic's Guide to Skiing

Books in the "Victim's Guide" series
($4.99 £2.99 paperback)

Award winning cartoonist Roland Fiddy sees the funny side to life's phobias, nightmares and catastrophes.

The Victim's Guide to the Dentist
The Victim's Guide to the Doctor
The Victim's Guide to Middle Age

Great Britain: Order these super books from your local bookseller or from Exley Publications Ltd, 16 Chalk Hill, Watford, Herts WD1 4BN. (Please send £1.30 to cover postage and packing on 1 book, £2.60 on 2 or more books.)